How I Mastered Looking Young

and

Staying Healthy Naturally

Alicia Lemourt-Hernandez

Balboa Press books may be ordered through booksellers or by contacting:

Balboa Press
A Division of Hay House
1663 Liberty Drive
Bloomington, IN 47403
www.balboapress.com
1 (877) 407-4847

Because of the dynamic nature of the Internet, any web addresses or links contained in this book may have changed since publication and may no longer be valid. The views expressed in this work are solely those of the author and do not necessarily reflect the views of the publisher, and the publisher hereby disclaims any responsibility for them.

The information, ideas, and suggestions in this book are not intended as a substitute for professional medical advice. Before following any suggestions contained in this book, you should consult your personal physician. Neither the author nor the publisher shall be liable or responsible for any loss or damage allegedly arising as a consequence of your use or application of any information or suggestions in this book.

Any people depicted in stock imagery provided by Thinkstock are models, and such images are being used for illustrative purposes only.
Certain stock imagery © Thinkstock.

ISBN: 978-1-5043-4628-3 (sc)
ISBN: 978-1-5043-4629-0 (e)

Library of Congress Control Number: 2015919733

Print information available on the last page.

Balboa Press rev. date: 01/04/2016

BALBOA
PRESS
A DIVISION OF HAY HOUSE

CONTENTS

DEDICATION

This book is dedicated to my late mother, Rita, who was a great inspiration and role model for me. It is also dedicated to my husband Bob for his great support, encouragement, and love; to my son Gabriel; mother-in-law Consuelo; and brother-in-law David for their caring love and understanding.

I love you all, and God bless you!

ACKNOWLEDGMENTS

I would like to acknowledge Robert Hernandez, my dear husband, for his love, encouragement, and support. You made writing this book so much easier by being the best editor and technical support person a writer could ever have.

Perla Valdes, I extend my deepest gratitude for caring so much and sharing your wisdom and extremely good advice.

Cynthia Better, thank you for caring so much and being a very special friend.

Lisa Cougil, thank you for being there for me through tough times. Thank you for giving me a great gift, the book *You Can Heal Your Life* by Louise L. Hay in 1995.

The late Betty Lux, thank you for being my closest long-time and devoted friend.

Charles W. Creamer, Ph.D., thank you for giving me the encouragement to write this book.

INTRODUCTION

My story begins one beautiful day when I was about fourteen years old. I was talking to my mother about aging. She told me that the women in our family tended to gain some weight as they got older, especially around the hips, which was normal. I told her that I was not going to be one of them. I decided right then and there to find ways to stay slim and always look younger than my age. I went against the common belief that as we age, it is normal to gain weight, look old, and get sick.

Obviously getting older is unavoidable, but what if you can slow down the aging process by natural means and always look younger than your age? Wouldn't that be a great accomplishment? Add to that staying healthy. I made a decision early in my life to work on always looking younger than my real age. You see, I also believe that our health is one of the most important things in our lives. We can find happiness by doing things that we enjoy the most, but how much happier could we be if we could maintain our health?

I believe in taking preventive measures. Why wait for a problem to occur, that you then have to try to fix, if it could have been prevented in the first place?

Slowing down the aging process and staying healthy is possible, and in the following pages, I will tell you how I have been able to accomplish this so far in my life.

Our health begins in our minds and in our nutrition. One can enjoy life without overindulgence. As a young woman, I used to love to go dancing with friends and drink very moderately because I always wanted to be in control of my actions. Moderation, I believe, is one of the keys to having good health. Everything mentioned in this book is based on my own personal experiences and the information I have provided applies to both men and women.

The main reason I am writing this book is to convey a very important message. The message is there is a way to stay looking young while maintaining your health at the same time. Every now and then, I would run into or visit old friends. Whenever most of my friends saw me after a long time apart, they would ask me what I was doing in order to stay looking so young at my age. I have also experienced the same question from some of the clients at work. Whenever they ask me if I have children and I respond by saying that I have a thirty-two-year-old son, they looked at me with disbelief.

I enjoy helping people. If my message can help others improve their lives in some way, then I have succeeded in accomplishing my goal!

CHAPTER 1. HAIR

Throughout my life, I have researched and tried different products with the goal of maintaining my health, looking young, and keeping my hair healthy. As I grow older, the hair has been one of the most challenging tasks to maintain. When my menopause started, I lost a lot of my hair. It was scary. For many of us, maintaining our hair is a task that one needs to work on consistently. There are those lucky individuals who seem not to be affected by hormonal changes or age. There are various causes of hair loss, but the two I believe that affected me most were hormonal imbalance and stress. I will share with you what I have tried and what has worked for me.

There are so many products that claim to be the best, but not all of them seem to work as advertised. Always use a good organic shampoo without harsh ingredients—or at least one that contains natural ingredients, examples will be provided later in this chapter. But that is not all. You also need good nutrition. I have tried various supplements. Again, not all are the same. In my research, I found that it is a good idea to use a product that inhibits the production of DHT. What is DHT? Well, when the hormone testosterone is combined with an enzyme in our bodies called 5-alpha reductase, it becomes dihydrotestosterone (DHT). This hormone attacks the roots of our hair and causes the follicles to shrink and the hair to fall out. I will provide a product that will inhibit the production of DHT later in this chapter.

Another cause of hair loss is poor blood circulation to the scalp, which inhibits the flow of necessary nutrients to the hair roots. This can be caused by stress, which then results in tension of the neck muscles. Every so often I get a massage to help to ease stress, as well as take a day off from work.

Hair is at its most fragile state when wet. Therefore, be gentle in handling it. Try not to overprocess your hair too often with chemical products such as those associated with coloring, highlighting, relaxing, and perming. If you do, make sure that you apply a weekly treatment containing protein and moisturizing agents to prevent any hair breakage.

Repeated chemical services can contribute to hair breakage because the chemicals used in the process raise the hair's pH level, making it more alkaline. But what is pH? The term *pH* means "potential hydrogen." The pH levels are measured on a scale ranging from 0 to 14, where 7 is neutral. Levels below 7 are considered acidic, and levels above 7 are considered alkaline. Our hair and skin have an average pH level of 5 on this scale.

Chemical services raise the pH level of the hair. As a result of over processing, your hair will become dry and brittle, and breakage can occur. Later in this chapter, I will provide you with the product to use that will help with this condition.

My Current Hair Regimen

I. Scalp-Cleansing Oil:

I use Mirta de Perales (N) Treatment Oil, which can be used on normal-to-oily scalps. If you have a dry scalp, there is also an (S) Treatment Oil that you can use. These are not regular oils. These are great products. They cleanse the scalp, help the follicles to stay clean, and help the hair to stay strong and not fall out. I cover my scalp with it for about fifteen minutes before every shampoo as per the product's instructions. I massage it with a little bit of water to create some lather, and then I rinse it. I then follow this treatment with an organic shampoo or one that contains natural ingredients. These oils can be purchased on the web at www.amazon.com.

I use 2Chic Brazilian Keratin & Argan Oil Ultra-Sleek Shampoo by Giovanni that contains organic ingredients. I purchase it at Whole Foods. It is very good and leaves my hair very soft and shiny. You may also choose any other brand. Just make sure it contains natural and organic ingredients and no parabens. Parabens are preservatives used to avoid spoilage. I prefer to play it safe and use paraben-free products to avoid various skin irritations such as dermatitis and other allergic reactions.

I have also used Mill Creek Botanicals Biotin Shampoo Therapy Formula, which contains natural and organic ingredients. It is good for oily scalps. This shampoo can be purchased at any local Vitamin Shoppe store. Avoid harsh detergents whenever possible.

I also use a cleansing shampoo to get rid of buildup in the hair. I use Neutrogena Shampoo Anti-Residue Formula every two or three weeks. It leaves the hair very clean and removes all the residues left from conditioners and styling aids.

II. Conditioner:

If you have an oily scalp, do not apply conditioners to it. It will stimulate more oils. Just use a little bit on your hair, then rinse well. If you have a dry scalp, apply the conditioner all over your scalp and hair, leave it on for a few minutes, then rinse.

If you have dry hair, a good conditioner to use is Porosity Control Corrector & Conditioner made by Roux. Although it is not organic, it is still an exceptional product because it corrects your hair's pH level. This is a great product for chemically treated hair. It can be purchased at Sally Beauty Supply or on the web at www.amazon.com.

I am using 2Chic Brazilian Keratin & Argan Oil Ultra-Sleek Conditioner by Giovanni. It contains organic ingredients and is sold at Whole Foods.

III. Treatment:

It is advisable to do a deep-conditioning treatment weekly if you have extremely damaged hair. Once your hair is in a better state, you can then minimize the treatment frequency to monthly. Your hair will tell you whether it is healthy or not if you pay attention to it. This can be determined by the way it feels, how it looks, and its manageability.

Hair texture ranges between fine, medium, and coarse, and wave patterns range between straight, wavy, curly, and very tightly curled. All hair wave patterns are beautiful. The key is to learn how to handle your own. I have worked with all hair wave patterns and textures.

I personally use Nutrafix Hair Reconstructor by Giovanni. It is a deep-conditioning treatment. For extremely damaged hair, you can add a bit of conditioner to it to intensify the treatment. You then should wrap your head with a wet, hot towel—or use clear microwave plastic wrap—to keep your scalp warm; this will promote better absorption of the treatment. Depending on the condition of your hair, you can leave the treatment on between fifteen to thirty minutes. The worse it is, the longer you should treat it. You can purchase this product at Whole Foods.

IV. Supplements and Other Treatments:

I experienced hair loss due to hormonal changes during menopause. I have tried various products, and I have tested them for quality and results. Some are better than others.

I originally started using Hair Essentials Dietary Supplement (hair vitamins), which contains Chinese herbs, in September of 2011 with good results. My hair stopped falling out. The hair vitamins can be purchased on the web at www. naturalwellbeing.com.

However, I decided to continue my research and found yet another excellent product that I started using in September of 2013. I tested it by itself, and I am still using it. It also passed my test! It is called Poly Gro (Procyanidin). It is a high-potency topical solution that is applied to the scalp twice a day—once in the morning and once in the evening—along with a bit of massage to the scalp. There is also a capsule called Apple Polyphenols (Apple Poly). Both of these products are made from apples. They inhibit the enzyme 5-alpha-reductase which converts testosterone to DHT. They are all natural, and I am having fantastic results. New hairs are growing, giving me more hair density, and it is nice to use products that really work without side effects! These two products can be purchased on the web at www.applepoly.com/healthyhair. I recommended this product to various friends, and they are also having very good results.

Since Hair Essentials Dietary Supplement and both Apple Poly products are different, I recently decided to try them together to see what would happen. On February 27, 2015, I began using both product lines. I take one Apple Poly capsule daily along with the recommended dosage of Hair Essentials (three capsules). As a result of doing so, I continue to experience no hair loss, and abundance of new hair growth. A small amount of daily hair loss is normal; however, an excessive amount is not.

I am also currently using a laser comb for about twelve minutes twice a week, running the laser beam over my scalp. This device is FDA approved to stimulate the hair follicles and promote hair growth. Using the laser comb can achieve enhanced results.

If you blow-dry your hair, which most of us do, you should apply a protecting spray right before blow-drying, such as Keratin & Green Tea Restructurizer made by ApHogee. This product provides hair care and protection against heat. It can be purchased at Sally Beauty Supply or any other beauty supply store.

On the average, hair usually grows a half an inch per month. You will need to be patient and consistent when using a hair improvement regimen in order to see results. The condition of my hair has gotten better. However, I still feel that there is room for improvement, thus I continue to work on it.

Hair Progression Images

Please refer to the before and after progression images located at the end of this chapter. These images will show you my hair progression over time as a result of proper diet and use of the products I mentioned in this chapter.

Before Progression Images

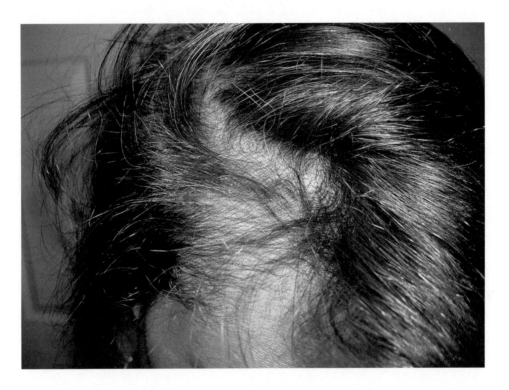

Taken on 03/29/10. This photo represents the recession
area on the top right side of my hairline.

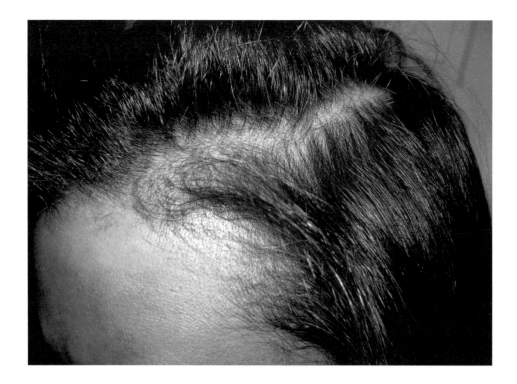

Taken on 03/29/10. This photo represents the recession area on the left side of my hairline.

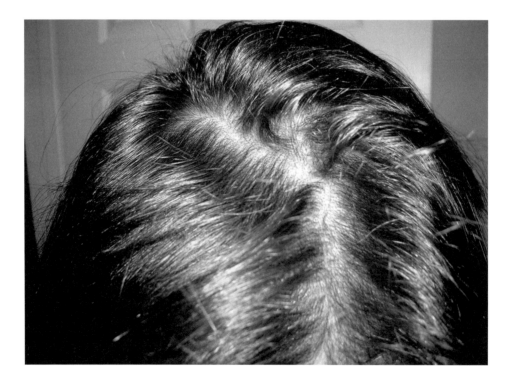

Taken on 03/29/10. This photo represents the recession area on the left side of my hairline.

After Progression Images

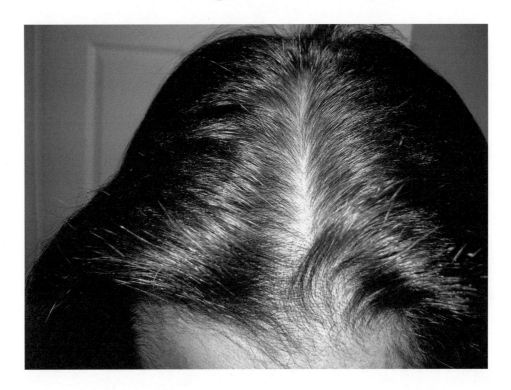

Taken on 04/05/12. This photo represents the
thinning area on the top of my head.

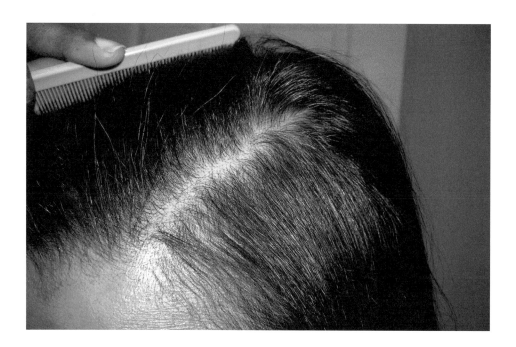

Taken on 08/20/12. This photo represents the recession area on the left side of my hairline.

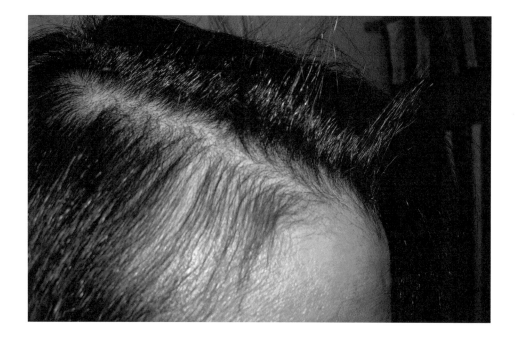

Taken on 08/20/12. This photo represents the recession area on the right side of my hairline.

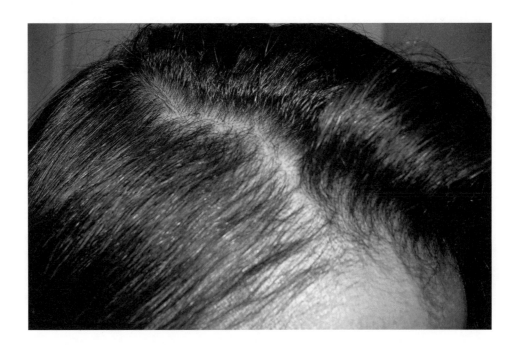

Taken on 11/04/13. This photo represents the recession area on the right side of my hairline. I started using Apple Poly hair products on 09/27/13.

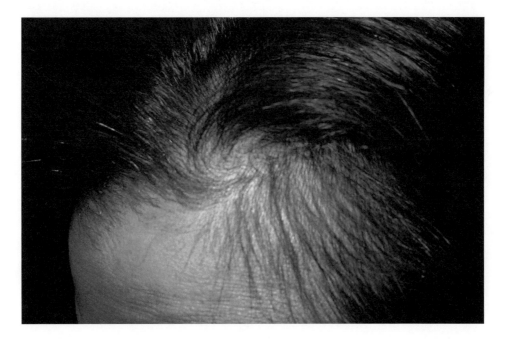

Taken on 11/20/13. This photo represents the recession area on the left side of my hairline.

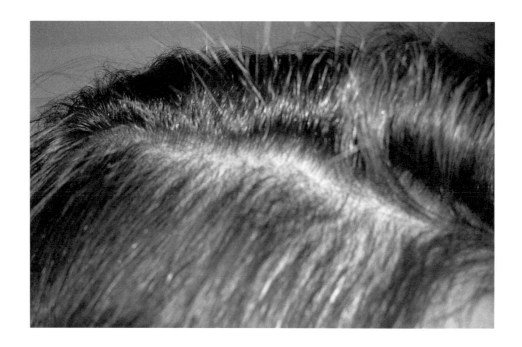

Taken on 02/09/14. This photo represents the recession area on the right side of my hair line. This is four and a half months after using Apple Poly.

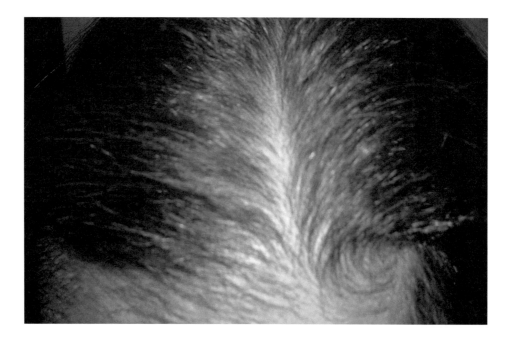

Taken on 01/04/15. This photo represents the thinning area on the top of my head.

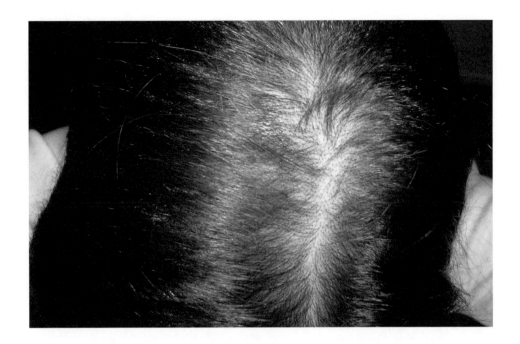

Taken on 01/04/15. This photo represents the thinning area on the top of my head.

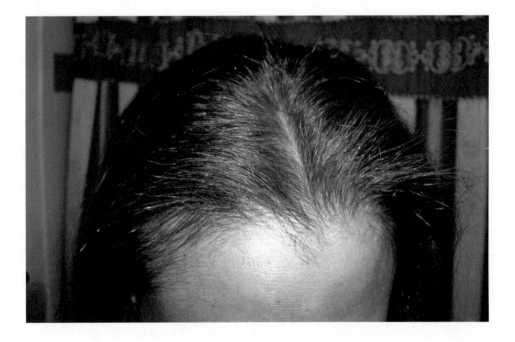

Taken on 05/24/15. This photo represents the area on the top of my head. This is approximately three months after having started using both Apple Poly and Hair Essentials products.

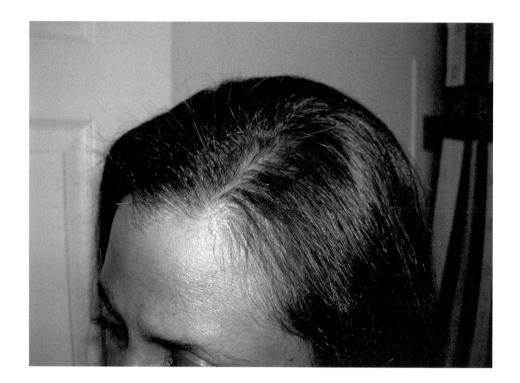

Taken on 05/24/15. This photo represents a view of the top left side of my head.

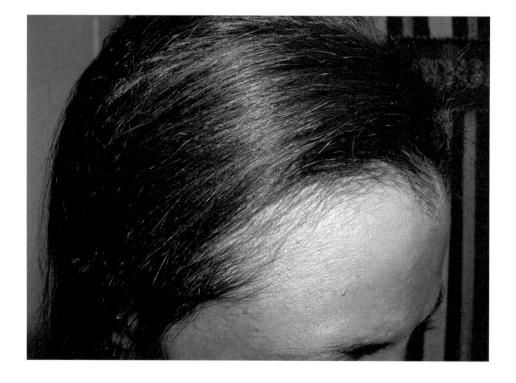

Taken on 05/24/15. This photo represents a view of the top right side of my head.

CHAPTER 2. SKIN (FACE/BODY)

It's not only important what you use on your skin but also what you eat and take as supplements.

A great supplement for your skin is collagen. Our bodies produce collagen, but as we reach the age of thirty-five and older, its production decreases. As a result, we experience wrinkles and sagginess of the skin. Collagen (a protein) is an important building block in maintaining tight skin. It is also beneficial toward joint flexibility.

I currently eat foods that help my body to produce collagen naturally. For example, I eat dark green vegetables such as kale, spinach, and broccoli. You can also eat collard greens, asparagus, Brussels sprouts, and cauliflower. They all contain vitamins A and C. Vitamin C is essential for collagen production. Some of the fruits that are rich in vitamin C include kiwi, oranges, lemons, strawberries, and pink grapefruit. Pink grapefruit contains a high percentage of the recommended dietary allowance of vitamin C and it also contains vitamin A. It contains a carotenoid called lycopene, which happens to be a potent antioxidant. Kiwi is a major source of vitamins C and E and is also very low in sugar. Studies have shown that kiwi improves skin appearance. Other fruits containing this antioxidant are apricots, papaya, and tomatoes. I eat a variety of these fruits.

I like to make a fruit cocktail from fresh fruits, which taste great. I include, for example, pineapple, pink grapefruit, orange, kiwi, green apple, strawberries, and papaya. You can also make it differently by replacing the pineapple and orange with apricots and keep everything else the same. You can also add pears and blueberries. Just mix and match.

Other ways to maintain healthy skin are to avoid smoking, drink plenty of water, and get enough sleep. If you drink alcohol, it should be done moderately. I drink between six to eight glasses of spring water a day and get about seven hours of sleep a night. Drinking plenty of water helps to keep our skin hydrated. I do not drink any soda. Moderate sleep and rest helps you to look young. I also make sure to protect my face from the sun using a moisturizer that contains sun screen with SPF of 30. Overexposure to sunlight may cause skin cancer and make you develop dark spots.

I have learned that we need to have both essential and nonessential amino acids. Amino acids are considered building blocks of proteins. However, our bodies do not produce the essentials. Therefore, we need to acquire them from food or supplemental sources. Foods such as lentils, peanuts, eggs, and chicken, which I also eat, are a good source. There are other sources as well.

The nonessential amino acids support tissue growth and repair. Our bodies are able to produce those. We also need antioxidants to help neutralize free radicals that can attack the skin cells. I take 500mg of grape seed extract in order to accomplish this.

We also need to use good-quality makeup products on a regular basis in order to maintain skin integrity. After having used and tested various products on the market and having returned some of them due to allergic reactions, thus far, the product line that I have used that has given me the best results has been Juice Beauty.

Face

Daily Regimen:

Morning:

My current regimen includes some of the *Juice Beauty* product line. These products are certified organic and they work well with my skin. I wash my face with the Cleansing Milk. Lately, I have been using the Juice Beauty Exfoliating Cream on a daily basis using a wash cloth. It is very good and leaves the skin feeling very soft. I then spray the Juice Beauty Hydrating Mist, followed by Juice Beauty Antioxidant Serum on my face and neck. This serum helps diminish the appearance of fine lines and wrinkles. This is followed by the Juice Beauty Nutrient Moisturizer. It contains rich antioxidants that hydrates and replenishes the skin. For my eyes, I apply Juice Beauty Soothing Eye Concentrate Cream. Use a very small amount of this product. It will be enough for both eyes. Apply it using your ring finger. By doing so, you will not apply too much pressure. Be gentle and do not stretch the skin, or sagginess can develop over time. As a sunscreen, I use Replenishing Solar Defense SPF30 by MyChelle Dermaceuticals. I purchase these products at Whole Foods.

Never wash your face with regular soap. Soaps contain detergents that are harsh for your facial skin, stripping it of its natural oils.

I also use some of the Bobbi Brown makeup line, such as the pressed powder and blush to name a few. They are very nice and you can purchase them at Macy's.

Night:

At night, I use the Cleansing Milk for cleansing my face with a wash cloth. Afterward, I apply the same serum and moisturizer used in the morning, and then I also apply a few drops of jojoba oil. Jojoba oil is a very thin oil that easily penetrates the skin as opposed to just laying on top of it. I have used it throughout my lifetime. If you have oily skin, do not use jojoba oil. Jojoba oil can be purchased at any health food store.

Juice Beauty has a Green Apple Age Defy organic solution product line for correcting and reducing dark spots as well as discoloration. It is excellent. I recently decided to try the collection kit and experienced positive results after just a few weeks. My skin is looking brighter and the few spots I have been trying to remove for a while are becoming less noticeable. Therefore, I am using less liquid foundation. I love it! According to their suggested instructions, individuals with sensitive skin should not use this line. My skin is sensitive but not highly sensitive, so I decided to try them cautiously. I have not experienced any negative reactions thus far. I plan to go back to the regular product line after I attain my intended goal. These products can be purchased directly at www.juicebeauty.com.

Weekly Regimen:

For many years I have been using Buf-Puf facial sponges to exfoliate my skin. Exfoliation is a process that helps to remove all dead skin cells. Be gentle when using the sponge. I use the Buf-Puf Gentle Facial Sponge. You can use this sponge with your favorite cleanser and gently massage your face and neck using a circular motion. Rinse the sponge well and let it dry after each use. I am currently using this sponge with Juice Beauty Exfoliating Cream.

A clay mask I like to use is called Indian Healing Clay made by Aztec Secret Health & Beauty, LTD. I like to use it on Sundays when I have more time. It is a strong mask. It removes dirt, impurities, and tightens up your facial pores. I prepare a small spoonful and add a capful of organic apple cider vinegar, a little water, and about five to ten drops of jojoba oil. If you have oily skin, do not add the jojoba oil. I mix it and create a soft paste, which I then apply to my face and neck with an applicator brush. You can also use your fingers. Make sure to avoid the eye area. As it dries, you will feel a very strong tightening sensation. I remove it after fifteen to twenty minutes with warm water and a wash cloth. Read the product instructions. The skin can become a bit pink; however, it goes away after about a half hour. I then apply the Juice Beauty Hydrating Mist, which tones and refreshes. I then massage a bit of jojoba oil and apply the Juice Beauty Nutrient Moisturizer. Your skin will feel very refreshed. I purchase the mask at Whole Foods.

When selecting your products, always check the expiration date. You do not want to use products that have already expired.

Eyelashes/Eyebrows

As we age, some of us experience thinning of our eyelashes and eyebrows. There are various products on the market today to help restore them.

I am currently using Adonia Lash Alive and Adonia Brow Revive made by Adonia Organics with very good results. Both of these are good for sensitive skin like mine. They contain organic ingredients that are not harmful.

You need to be consistent when using these products in order to see results. It definitely has worked for me. It is best to apply the products and let them dry before using a color pencil around the eyes and eyebrows. I do this to protect the eye lashes and the eyebrows from any chemicals in the pencils or similar makeup products. Limit the use of mascara. If you use it, use a good brand. Sometimes those products tend to make lashes and brows fall out. So make sure to create a barrier at the base before applying any color pencil or eye shadow.

Another method that I have tried is using the same Poly Gro liquid, used on the scalp for hair growth, on my eyebrows. Use the dropper applicator that comes in the package very carefully. You only need about three drops. So make sure the dropper only has a small amount of the liquid, otherwise you might squeeze too much and the liquid could run into your eyes. Place one drop at the beginning area of the brows, one in the center, and the last toward the end of the brow. Use your index finger to spread the solution throughout the eyebrow. Massage by pressing down, holding the position, and applying pressure in a circular motion. Keep doing this throughout the brow. Do not rub back and forth or you might cause some of the brow hair to fall out. Try this method for a month and evaluate your results. Remember that it takes time for hair to grow.

Facial Progression Images

Please refer to the before and after progression facial skin images at the end of this chapter. These images will show you my facial skin progression over a month's time as a result of using the Juice Beauty products I mentioned in this chapter. If the results you see here were for only one month, could you imagine the results after having used these products for a longer period of time?

Before Progression Images

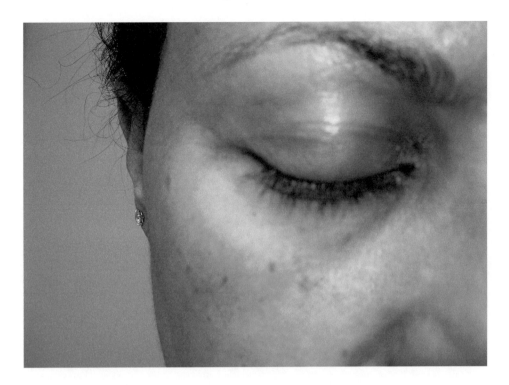

Taken on 04/22/15. This photo represents a view of
the area under my right eye and cheek.

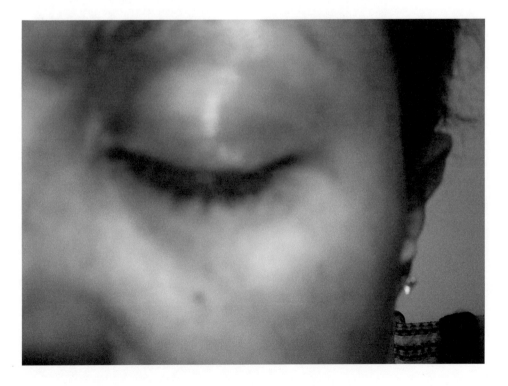

Taken on 04/22/15. This photo represents a view of
the area under my left eye and cheek.

After Progression Images

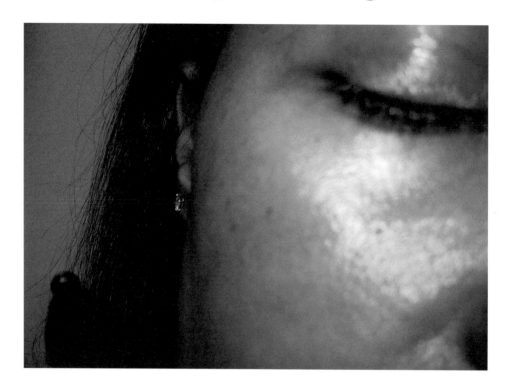

Taken on 05/24/15. This photo represents a view of the area under my right eye and cheek. This is about one month after using the Juice Beauty products.

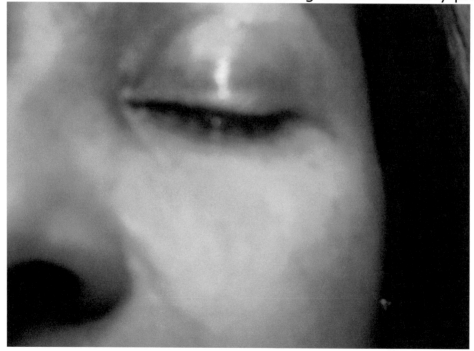

Taken on 05/24/15. This photo represents a view of
the area under my left eye and cheek.

Body

For my body I use Buf-Puf double-sided body sponge and Dr. Bronner's Hemp Pure Castile Liquid Soap (there are various fragrances). It can be purchased on the web from www.drugstore.com, www.drbronner.com, and at Vitamin Shoppe, Whole Foods, and other stores. At times, I also use conventional bar soap to minimize allergic skin reactions when I am not able to use Dr Bronner's liquid soap and to minimize the cost. Having used Buf-Puf throughout my life has helped me maintain skin that is consistently soft by removing dead cells, which create unwanted skin tones.

Right after taking a shower and drying I apply Aquaphor, a medicated ointment that helps maintain moisture throughout my body. I make sure to apply a bit under the arm pit and create a barrier before applying deodorant. I believe this helps minimize the amount of chemical that can enter the body through the pores under the arms. Remember, many deodorants contain aluminum chlorohydrate. I have done this throughout my life. Aquaphor is good for both men and women. My husband loves how my skin feels!

The Bacteria Skin Infection Story

I would like to tell you a story about my son. In 2011, he was having major challenges due to a staph bacteria skin infection that was developing on a monthly basis. For example, a small pimple would develop and it would grow inward underneath the skin. It would become very large, about two-and-a-half inches in diameter and deep; very painful. It was unbelievable!

We went to the hospital emergency room various times. Pimples would grow back in various parts of his body: for example, one time on the leg, another time on the thigh, then in the back and stomach areas. Each time antibiotics would be administered, but it would return after a month or so. I did not know what to do to help my son, and I was hoping the doctors would find the cure. The doctors did what they could. Unfortunately, there is no cure for this condition; only antibiotics to control it. The infection was proven to be MRSA, which is contagious, and he was isolated in the hospital.

While in the hospital he asked me to bring his laptop computer. He decided to do research to learn more about this condition and hopefully find a way to eliminate it. Not only did he find out that many people suffered from the same condition, but he also found a way to control it. He contacted the company using his cell phone; spoke to a representative who was very helpful in order to learn additional information. He gave me information to read. At that point we were desperate and hopeful at the same time. We decided to order the product. We had nothing to lose since there was nothing else that would help him anyway.

It took a couple of months for the product to start working. The pimples would develop smaller and would eventually disappear. The product is called Phenomenal. It's been about four years since he started taking this product, and now he takes less of it and pimples have not developed. I am so grateful that this product exists. This product can be purchased on the web at www.phenomenalwater.com.

CHAPTER 3. OVERALL HEALTH

I have always been interested in my overall health. I believe we become the product of how we think, what we eat, and what we do. Healthy meals will result in healthy bodies. Unhealthy foods eaten throughout your life will give you a higher chance of incurring ailments at a younger age. If you smoke and drink alcohol excessively, that will also increase the chances of developing various diseases such as COPD (chronic obstructive pulmonary disease), cardiovascular disease, lung cancer, liver problems, and more. I have always said, "Why create a problem for myself health-wise?" There are enough challenges that we must face in our lives, why create more? It is a fact that we are not going to be on this earth forever. However, that is no reason to create more problems that will shorten our lifespan, not to mention the suffering that we can experience from these ailments. If by chance an ailment develops is one thing, but to create it by committing unhealthy actions and being in denial about it and thinking that it is never going to happen to you seems a bit foolish, wouldn't you think so?

My mother always used to tell me to take care of myself. Any ailment you have when you are young usually becomes worse as you age. I lived through a very painful experience seeing how much my mother suffered from asthma toward the end of her life. She had asthma since childhood, even though she never smoked. Her asthma was controlled throughout her lifetime. It became worse as she grew older, and she lived to be almost ninety-three. She passed away four days before her ninety-third birthday. She lived the best she could under the circumstances and succeeded. She taught me to do things in moderation and to create peace within myself and with those around me.

Our bodies are susceptible to deficiencies, wear and tear. At times we need supplements to help restore the balance within our bodies. Any of our organs can malfunction or have a deficiency.

I think one key is prevention. The other is to maintain a good mental attitude by resolving the uncomfortable situations in our lives that give us high levels of stress. Stress must be eliminated or at least minimized. I believe stress is not a disease. In my opinion, it is a state of mind caused by someone or something that makes us uncomfortable due to actions or lack of actions and/or disagreements. You can read more about this in chapter 4.

I started doing some reading in reference to the relationship between the food we eat and our health. I told my husband about the information that I found. Based on what we read, we needed to make some changes. At first he became concerned and asked me, "What are we going to eat then?"

What about the foods we are used to eating? Most people do not like to make changes, especially in their diet. I told him we just needed to substitute some of the foods we were eating with those containing less harmful ingredients. It was a wake-up call in reading the ingredient labels on the boxes and cans we had at home. We learned exactly what to look for.

The bottom line is to start eating more organic foods. This means eliminating pesticides on fruits, vegetables, and grains. The same pertains to growth hormones in meats. Just remember, whatever the animals eat we also consume. This holds true for poultry, eggs, farm-raised cows (red meat), their milk, and farm-raised fish. The percentage of chemicals, preservatives, and pesticides currently found in conventional foods are deemed not to be harmful for human consumption by the US Food and Drug Administration (FDA). However, it is my opinion that if one repeatedly eats conventional foods containing these types of chemicals over a long period of time, it could create various types of harmful diseases such as cancer, tumors, hair loss, and so forth.

You can recognize organic versus conventional vegetables and fruits by looking at the first digit of the four- or five-digit product lookup (PLU) code sticker. For example, the number 9 is organic (preferred). The number 4 is conventional, which means it was grown using chemicals, such as pesticides or herbicides. The number 8 is genetically modified (GMO) food, which is not labeled all the time (stay away from those). There is another code, 3, that is still unclear as to whether it is conventional or genetically modified. However, let me tell you a story of what happened to me.

In 2014, I purchased a papaya that had the number 3 as the first digit of the PLU code. The papaya looked very appealing in color and texture. The next morning I prepared my usual smoothie using a piece of the papaya. About one hour later I felt nauseous and had some sort of allergic reaction, which caused me to sneeze incessantly. I tried again for another two days and had the same reaction. Afterward, I decided to take a break from eating papaya. Months later, I decided to try again. This time I happened to purchase a papaya with a PLU code beginning with the number 4 (conventional). I was pleasantly surprised that I had no reaction. Therefore, I continued adding it to my smoothies with no fear.

In 2015, I was in a hurry and purchased another papaya without looking at the PLU code. The papaya looked good to me. An hour after having drunk my smoothie that included the papaya, I was at my morning meeting at work. I again began to sneeze incessantly and felt very nauseous. When I got home after work, I took a look at the PLU code and to my surprise I noticed that it began with the number 3.

In conclusion, stay away from fruits and vegetables with PLU codes beginning with a 3, as well as those starting with an 8.

People are accustomed to buying conventional produce because it is more available in the marketplace and it costs less than the organic kind. In recent years, organic produce has become more available, thus making it easier to purchase. When purchasing conventional produce you can use a fruit and vegetable wash solution such as Trader Joe's Fruit & Vegetable Wash, or other like products that help to remove pesticides, waxes, and chemicals from the outer skin of your conventional produce. Using this wash helps to minimize your chemical intake. The alternative and best solution is to buy organic produce, especially when the skin is eaten. Those are more expensive but contain no chemicals.

The Mammogram Story

In November of 2008, I went for my regularly scheduled mammogram. The mammogram showed that I had calcifications in my left breast and that more tests had to be done. I was very upset and concerned after learning this, although I tried to keep calm. The hospital scheduled a biopsy to be performed. After waiting for a few days that seemed to be forever, I was told that I was fine and that no cancer was detected. However, I needed to schedule another mammogram six months later.

I decided to do more in-depth research that resulted in my decision to cleanse my body and learn more about maintaining my overall health. In my research, I learned that it was important to eliminate heavy metals from our bodies. Heavy metals, such as mercury and lead, can lead to a number of major illnesses. Mercury, for example, is extremely toxic. It is found in our bodies via what we eat. Silver dental fillings are also a source of mercury.

When you eat certain types of fish like tuna, you can end up with a mercury build-up in your body, especially if you eat an abundance of it. Foods that contain high fructose corn syrup, unfortunately, can also contain traces of mercury due to the way they are processed. Try to avoid foods containing this additive.

I also learned that the herb cilantro possesses the ability of removing heavy metals from our bodies. So I gathered ingredients from various sources and created the following recipe:

- Cilantro - organic   1 bunch
- Extra virgin olive oil   1 cup
- Garlic - organic   6 cloves
- Lemon - organic   1 squeezed

- Turmeric - organic   1/2 teaspoon
- Sea salt   to taste
- Ground flaxseed   2/3 cup
- Ginger root (no skin)   1/4 cup

You can use a blender or the NutriBullet. Blend it to make a paste, store it in small containers, and put them in the freezer. Leave one small container in the refrigerator. I would take one tablespoon of this paste daily and drink water afterward.

After having used this recipe for six months, I went for another mammogram nine months after my initial one and was told that the results were normal and to schedule a regular yearly visit. I was ecstatic and really took very seriously the idea of eating more organic foods and just eating healthily.

Daily Routine

I drink two glasses of spring water as soon as I get up in the morning and one more after my twenty minutes of exercise. Altogether, I drink a total of six to eight glasses of spring water throughout the day. Moderate exercise helps maintain our overall health. It provides healthier heart function and more energy. You burn up the excess sugar in the bloodstream, which can possibly contribute to the development of diabetes.

I had a blood test done in May of 2014 and my hemoglobin A1C level was 6.0, which indicated that I fell in the category for an increased risk of diabetes. After my doctor reviewed the results of my blood test, he felt that there was no need for any major concern. I still did research on how to improve sugar levels in the blood and learned that the liver plays a major role in maintaining healthy sugar levels. Combined with a proper diet, it is possible that the hemoglobin A1C level would then normalize (lower) depending on one's physical anatomy. Make sure to have an annual checkup, request to receive a copy of the results, and pay attention to the results. Monitor the areas that are out of range from your blood test results and discuss them with your doctor or nutritionist. The nutritionist can then develop a proper diet for you.

After having done some research, I learned that kale has great nutritional value. It acts as an antioxidant and anti-inflammatory agent. It helps to detoxify the body and blocks cancer cell growth. It also helps lower cholesterol. It is high in fiber, vitamins, and minerals. It can cleanse the liver and consequently help lower sugar levels. I decided to test it. I stopped adding sugar to my teas and stopped eating sweets. I added kale to my daily diet as described in the Breakfast section below. Kale might interfere with calcium absorption, so it should be taken separately from any high-calcium foods or supplements.

I included kale in my daily smoothies for four months. In September of 2014, I did another blood test and to my surprise the hemoglobin A1C went down to 5.7 and I lost ten pounds without trying. I worked on gaining a few pounds back. Amazing!

One can cure or improve many ailments with proper nutrition, common sense, and properly administered natural supplements. My husband and I both take Nature's Plus Source of Life Gold Liquid multivitamins and minerals. I believe liquid supplements are better absorbed by our bodies. All other supplements I take are mostly in capsule form.

Always read the contents on the containers and compare their ingredients. Ensure that sugar and sodium levels are low for various health reasons, including yeast outgrowth. I learned that we need to eat some raw foods, not just cooked, so keep it balanced. Try to stay away from junk food. Although they taste good, the results are devastating when consumed long term.

I usually do my basic grocery shopping at Trader Joe's and Whole Foods. If you like to eat certain types of "fun" food, such as tortilla chips, you can purchase them at both of these stores. They are tasty and healthier because they contain healthy ingredients.

Breakfast

I drink a smoothie every morning for breakfast. My basic smoothie consists of kale, three organic fruits, such as a small or half of a regular-size cored green apple, two strawberries, a small piece of papaya, a squeeze of a small slice of lemon, about twelve raw almonds (sometimes soaked overnight), organic almond milk, a teaspoon of chia seeds, a scoop of pea protein and a little spring water.

Other times I make a different smoothie using spinach, spirulina powder, or sun chlorella in a granulated form. They have great nutritional value. Sometimes I may also add one tablespoon of whole oat groats soaked overnight to my smoothie. If you are trying to decrease sugar levels, keep using the kale. To make my smoothie, I use the NutriBullet machine. It's fantastic and easy to use. It comes with a booklet with suggestions of what to make as well as different types of meals for overall health.

Sometimes I make a smaller smoothie and combine it with one slice of organic sprouted multigrain bread with an organic buttery spread or a no- nut spread made from golden peas. I sometimes like to change the fruits. I would mix a piece of pineapple, three strawberries, and a small pear, or add blueberries instead. You can also interchange with a piece of mango. It tastes great!

I also make smoothies with one carrot, one small apple, and one small beet, a slice of lemon with the peel, kale, a small piece of chopped-up ginger, and almond milk. There are many varieties that you can make.

Lunch

I vary my lunches. I either have leftovers from the night before, something like fish, organic mixed vegetables, or broccoli and a bit of quinoa. Other times I might have organic lentil soup or any other soup, most of the time packaged in a carton, although sometimes I may eat a soup from a can. I may eat a salad with organic salad mixed greens, which comes in a bag. I add radish, red onions, olives, a cooked beet; a bit of raw carrots, red peppers, or roasted red peppers from a glass jar. I might also add steamed broccoli or a bit of spinach. For the dressing, I prefer using lemon juice, extra virgin olive oil, a bit of sea salt, sprinkled organic garlic powder, and oregano. Once in a while I might use an organic light balsamic dressing. Lemon has many benefits, including helping to make our bodies more alkaline versus acidic. These are just some examples. You can use your own combination of vegetables to create a nice tasty lunch!

Snacks

For snacks, I like to eat raw walnuts and almonds containing no added sugar or salt coating. Our bodies do not need to process any extra sugar or salt. Excess salt can cause hardening of the arteries and water retention in your legs, especially as we age. We already know about the growing problem of diabetes in our country due to the increased consumption of sweets in our diets and the added sugar in processed foods.

Another tasty snack I enjoy eating is Trader Joe's Quinoa and Black Bean Tortilla Chips. They are low in salt and contain no sugar. I also enjoy having the Trader Joe's Fat Free Spicy Black Bean Dip with the chips.

At night I enjoy eating an orange or half a grapefruit or a pear a couple of hours after having dinner. They improve my bowel movements in the morning. You can also enjoy other fruits. From my research, it is of utmost importance that one has at least two bowel movements per day. If you have three, it is even better. The result will be a healthier colon. Lack of frequent bowel movements could cause the formation of putrefied matter in the colon, like a "traffic jam." As a result, this condition could contribute to illnesses such as colon cancer and diverticulitis. Most doctors suggest scheduling a colorectal exam (colonoscopy) at the age of fifty and every five years thereafter. I already had mine done with good results.

Dinner

I like to eat as much organic foods as possible along with conventional. I combine vegetables with ground turkey, organic chicken, or fish (such as wild caught salmon or Dover sole). I also eat brown rice (less processed) or quinoa, red or black beans, or lentils. You can mix and match. Other times we eat organic pasta with broccoli and organic pasta sauce. I believe eating healthy and in moderation. We try to mix proteins with vegetables, such as chicken or fish with vegetables. We also mix carbohydrates with vegetables, such as pasta with vegetables and pasta sauce. Both of these combinations make it easy for our stomachs to digest. Some of the oils and spices I use to prepare our foods are extra virgin olive oil, coconut oil, cumin, oregano, turmeric, parsley, garlic, onions, sea salt, ginger, basil, fennel seed, and rosemary. Most of the spices I use are organic.

Balancing Organic and Conventional Foods in Your Diet

I believe everyone should eat about 70 percent organic and about 30 percent conventional foods. Although it is healthy to eat organic food, you must also incorporate conventional food in your diet in order to avoid experiencing an allergic reaction. This happened to me in the past. At one point in time, I was eating only organic foods. I was at work one day and lunch was served during a meeting for all the employees. I decided to eat the food and experienced an allergic reaction. I became nauseous and developed a skin rash about a half hour later. I then realized that my body was not used to the conventional food any longer. Therefore, I decided to incorporate some conventional food in my diet to overcome this problem. Thus far, it has been working.

Alkaline and Acidic Foods

In my research, I also learned that eating foods that are alkaline helps to maintain better health. So it is a good idea to incorporate alkaline foods in our diet. For example, most green vegetables and sprouts are considered alkaline foods.

According to my research, bacteria, viruses, cancer, and yeast cannot live in an alkaline environment. I had an experience with my son's recurring staph infection and how we got rid of it as described in chapter 2 of this book. For additional details on alkaline foods, the web is a good source for identifying both alkaline and acidic foods, as well as the neutral ones. I feel that it is important to maintain a balance between all of them. The more we learn about how to maintain good health, the fewer the problems we shall encounter in the future as we grow older. I feel that if we use preventive measures we can avoid many health challenges that are common in our society.

About Sweets

Sugar is habit forming, but so is not having much sugar in our diets. I learned that it is important to cut down on the sugar intake, natural or synthetic. I ask myself, why is it that in our country we have such a high number of diabetics? I think it is due to a combination of reasons. We are a fast-moving society concerned most of the time with making money, paying bills, and we have high levels of stress caused by our jobs and personal lives. Most of the time people eat fast foods with soft drinks. If you take the time to look at the amount of sugar in those soft drinks and multiply it by the number of days that you are having those drinks, no wonder we end up having an overabundance of sugar in our bloodstream. And when you add processed foods that are also being consumed, they also turn into sugar.

What about the desserts that taste so good but have loads of sugar? Our bodies are not equipped to process that overabundance of sugar. This can result in diabetes or other ailments.

Once in a while, I believe it is fine to have something sweet. The problem starts when you have it consistently. Holidays are the roughest times. There is always an overabundance of sweets everywhere: at work, gifts, and so forth. What amazes me is that if you are not used to eating so many sweets, your body rejects the sugar after a while. I have experienced this myself. I choose not to buy any sugar or add any in what I consume. That is just my personal choice, and it is working quite well. By the way, my husband does not consume sugar either.

We need to eat a bit more *moderately and balanced*. We should cut down on the amount of cookies, cakes, ice cream, and similar sweets that we consume. Refer to the Daily Routine and Breakfast sections for suggested solutions. Look for the glycemic index chart on the web to determine sugar levels in foods.

Reference to Headaches

During the months of January and February of 2013, I experienced unusual headaches on a daily basis. At first, I attributed the headaches to the stress that I had been going through with my ill mother and work-related issues. In 2012, my mother had been hospitalized eight times. My stress level had been very high. I decided to learn the cause of my headaches, not just mask it with some pain killers. I used holistic liquid medicine, which helped, but the headaches would return. I do not take over-the-counter painkillers. I believe it is best to find the cause rather than just address the symptoms. Can you imagine how difficult it was having daily headaches and working under those conditions?

I said to myself: "Somehow the information will come and I will learn the cause of these headaches". Well, I received a book from American Botanicals, by Dr. Schulze, from whom I purchase holistic supplements from time to time. I did not purchase the book; it just came in the mail. This book was an eye opener. After I started reading it, I realized what was causing my headaches. It was due to an accumulation of toxins as well as stress. Due to working late hours and taking care of my mom, I would come home late very often. I did not have time to cook at home, so I was purchasing cooked conventional food and bringing it home for dinner. I believe one could eat out once in a while but not consistently, especially when you are accustomed to eating organic foods cooked at home.

I have been eating organic food at home for the past five years and only once or twice per week eating conventional food. I decided to test my theory. I needed to do a colon cleansing as the book suggested. I ordered the 5 Day Detox Program. In the meantime, I happened to have at home one of Dr. Schulze's products for the colon, Formula #1. I took three capsules after dinner. The next day I noticed that my headache was much better after having a bowel movement. I also learned that in order to avoid disease, we needed to have a clean colon. We should have a bowel movement half an hour to an hour after having a meal. Basically, we should go to the bathroom two to three times a day. We do not think about it, but it makes sense to maintain a clean colon, getting rid of all the waste and residues from everything we eat. Otherwise, this becomes toxic and can spread throughout our bodies, making us ill. I believe that not only do we need to eat quality food but we also need to clean our bodies from the inside out.

When the detox program package arrived, I used Formula #1 for two additional days and ate only salads and vegetables. About a month later, I visited a nutritionist who reviewed my current diet and supplements. I learned that I needed to complete my cleansing by drinking juices for three days and to stop eating chicken, lamb, beef and fish, which I did. My headaches went away as a result of using the colon cleansing Formula #1 and the three-day fasting using juices that I made. I experience a great relief!

Another product I use for eliminating headaches is a product called Migrastick, which is a small roll-on stick containing 100 percent pure and natural essential oils. It is applied to the forehead and temples when a headache begins and this helps to eliminate it. I purchase it at Vitamin Shoppe. Breathing deeply, inhaling and exhaling slowly also helps.

Cleansing/Detoxification Formulas

Upon further research, I also learned that chlorella, which is a sea algae, contains great nutritional value. For example, it can detoxify our bodies, by helping to eliminate pesticides and heavy metals. It is considered a "super food." I found Sun Chlorella to be a great product; it is all natural, easily absorbed by our bodies due to their processing methods specifically done by Sun Chlorella Corporation. It is a Japanese product. I add one individual packet of granules to my morning drink sometimes. I use the product for a couple of months then stop for a while and start again. It can be purchased at Vitamin Shoppe.

Another good product that I take at times is dandelion, which helps to cleanse your blood and liver. This is an herb that acts as a natural diuretic, (eliminates fluid retention). It helps improve kidney function as well as the pancreas. It also increases bile production. Bile is the digestive juice secreted by the liver and then stored by the gallbladder. You can either include it as an herb when making a juice or take it in a capsule form. If you suffer from gallbladder problems, speak to your nutritionist or doctor before using it. I also take at times milk thistle, but not at the same time with dandelion. Milk thistle protects the liver from free radicals. It has anticancer properties. It contains an ingredient called silymarin, which inhibits the formation of the enzyme COX-2. This enzyme produces a hormone which causes inflammation of the joints.

For Women During Menopause

Menopause became a life changing time for me. I started to lose my hair and had hot flashes at different times of the day and night. I did a lot of research to save my hair, control the hot flashes, and to try to feel better overall. I was able to find a way!

Menopause is a stage in our bodies' existence, just like puberty and adolescence. The world around us is in constant change, and we are a part of it. I decided to embrace menopause when it started rather than becoming stressed about it since I could not fight it.

During this phase of a woman's life, we go through some uncomfortable changes. They can be alleviated by using natural means to avoid the side effects that some prescription medications can produce.

I was able to control the hot flashes and sweats by using an herbal supplement called Lydia Pinkham Nutritional Supplement in a liquid form. My mother had told me about this natural supplement. It has been around since the 1800s, and it actually worked for me. You follow the instructions and find the amount that works best for you. I told my gynecologist about it. Since it was working, she agreed that I should continue using it rather than the recommended estrogen supplementation to alleviate the symptoms. This product can be found on the web or in some pharmacies. It is an over-the-counter, nonprescription product that really works! I used it for about two years and finally, I was done with my menopausal symptoms and have stopped taking it altogether. I feel very good now.

Improving Your Bone Structure

Years ago when my mother was alive, she was diagnosed with osteoporosis. This condition causes a loss of bone density and makes the bones become brittle and easy to fracture, especially if you fall. My mother was having problems with her hip. At times she felt a bit of a pain. The doctor told her that she needed to be hospitalized for a procedure that involved getting an injection containing a certain medicine in her hip. I was quite concerned with the whole procedure. I suggested that she try the calcium that I could get for her, and if it did not work, then do the procedure. She agreed. She started taking OsteoBalance by Pure Encapsulations following the dosage instructions. About six months later she had a bone density test done. The doctor asked her what she was doing, because her condition was definitely improving. She took the bottle to him and he told her to continue taking it. He was very surprised! My mother never had a fractured bone, although she had fallen a few times. I am currently using it myself.

Joint Discomfort

Due to a pair of skiing accidents I had in my younger years, every so often my knees would become stiff and painful. I had taken glucosamine for this condition. It helped somewhat. However, my doctor advised me not to take it for too long, as this could cause a high concentration of sugar levels. In July of 2014, I found a different supplement that I started having great results with. It is called Natural Joint by Greek Island Labs.

It promotes healthy joints and assists with overall flexibility and mobility. It contains a blend of thirty-seven natural ingredients and is a dietary supplement that actually works!

Respiratory Allergies and Eczema

I recently experienced a respiratory infection. My voice was hoarse and I had a runny nose. I was prescribed an antibiotic that I took for the required amount of time. Unfortunately, I was still feeling congested and had not completely recovered. I had symptoms similar to a respiratory allergy. I was prescribed a prednisone derivative. After having read about the side effects, I decided to do research in order to find something else that could help me without the side effects. I needed a natural anti-inflammatory supplement that would be useful in clearing my sinuses. I found a natural supplement called quercetin and bromelain made by Doctor's Best.

Quercetin is a bioflavonoid and bromelain is an enzyme. Both of these have anti-inflammatory properties and should be taken together to enhance absorption in the body. In order to obtain optimum results, I followed the instructions on the bottle and took 1,500 mg of quercetin and 750 mg of bromelain in divided dosages (two capsules, three times a day). After feeling better, I lowered my current dosage to two capsules, two times a day. You can decrease the amount according to your needs.

I have also taken two softgels of SinuCheck made by Enzymatic twice a day on and off, and only when necessary. This is a natural supplement containing Soledum-brand eucalyptus globulus oil extract. It is fantastic for clearing the sinuses.

As a result of taking both of these supplements, I am feeling greater relief with no side affects! Both of these products can be purchased at Vitamin Shoppe.

I currently have eczema on four of my fingers due to my job. While taking the quercetin and bromelain supplement, I noticed that my fingers became less swollen and the itchiness had diminished. I decided to read more about these supplements and discovered that they are also very effective for cases of eczema. I took the supplement for a few months until my overall sinus and eczema condition became much better, and then I decided to stop. A few weeks later, I noticed that the eczema on my fingers flared up again with major itchiness and swelling. Therefore, I decided to start taking the supplement again, resulting in major improvement. While taking this supplement, I also applied Aquaphor Healing Ointment made by Eucerin on my hands. Using this ointment will help to maintain some moisture to the affected area and provide relief for skin dryness and itchiness. This ointment should be applied several times a day in order to be effective. I always carry a small tube with me in my purse.

In addition to taking the quercetin and bromelain supplement, I am also taking OPtiMSM Best MSM made by Doctor's Best. Methylsulfonylmethane (MSM) is an organic sulfur compound found in animal and plant tissue. MSM is used for healing of injuries, cellular detoxification, hair, skin and nail nourishment, and in the reduction of pain and inflammation. The recommended dosage of MSM should be 2000 mg per day in divided dosages with meals. I was originally taking 1000 mg of MSM per day to heal the cracks in the skin on my fingers caused by the excess dryness from the eczema. However, I decided to increase the dosage to 2000 mg. As a result of having done so, not only did the skin cracking condition heal, but the eczema has improved significantly.

Eye Twitching Caused by Stress

I experienced twitching in my left eye caused by a combination of job stress and family-related issues. I felt very uncomfortable whenever I spoke to people at work, and my eye was constantly twitching. In order to relieve this condition, I used an herbal supplement that I purchased from American Botanicals by Dr. Schulze called Nerve. I took thirty drops of the Nerve supplement in two ounces of water at breakfast and at dinner time, followed by a glass of water. Then I increased the dosage to forty drops. It is best to increase the dosage gradually. When I began taking this supplement, I noticed that the twitching gradually decreased. After having taken this supplement for four days, the twitching went away completely! Thus, I stopped taking it.

Teeth and Gum Care

It is very important to incorporate flossing before brushing your teeth at night. I personally use Jason Powersmile Antiplaque & Whitening toothpaste. It is fluoride and sulfate free. You can purchase this toothpaste at Vitamin Shoppe. I personally believe that the fewer amounts of chemicals and additives a product contain, the better it is for one's overall health.

For my teeth and gums, I use Dr. Schulze's Tooth & Gum herbal formula made by American Botanical Pharmacy. I use it twice a month for maintenance. I apply it directly to my gums and teeth using a Q-tip cotton swab before going to bed. The most important thing is to brush and floss. My teeth and gums are very healthy as a result of doing so.

Throat and Tonsil Care

When I was a child in Cuba, I used to suffer from tonsillitis, and at times, bronchitis. My mother would give me cod liver oil to treat the bronchitis. After I arrived in the United States, during the winter months I would develop these same two symptoms. My mother took me to a physician in New Jersey near our home to have them treated. When he diagnosed my condition, he tried to avoid having surgery in order to save my tonsils. He explained that the tonsils were the body's first line of defense for trapping any incoming bacteria. He performed a culture in order to find the cause of the condition and properly treat it. When all was done, he prescribed me a certain type of vitamin to take that contained vitamin A. I took this vitamin for about six years in addition to a teaspoon of cod liver oil daily. As the years passed, my condition improved immensely. Combined with my current diet, I not only still have my tonsils but I do not suffer from tonsillitis any longer. Before resorting to surgery, we should do our utmost to get treatment for the condition to try to save the organ.

For my throat and tonsils, I have used Dr. Schulze's Throat & Tonsil herbal formula made by American Botanical Pharmacy. It comes in both a spray and dropper form and is very potent. Use this product per the bottle's instructions at the first sign of a sore throat. All of American Botanical Pharmacy products can be purchased on the web at www.herbdoc.com.

Managing Your Weight

An essential part of maintaining your overall health is by managing your weight. At the end of December of 2002, I made a new year's resolution to work on losing weight. At that time I weighed 137 pounds. In January of 2003, I began working out at home on a stationary machine doing cardiovascular exercises to lose weight and tone my muscles. By February of 2003, I weighed 134 pounds. I only lost three pounds and was very disappointed. Therefore, I gave up exercising all together.

In May of 2003, I weighed myself and weighed 136 pounds. I then decided to resume my exercise program. I was unhappy with the way my clothes fitted; they were too tight. I went through various weight gains and losses exercising on my own and stopping in between. These lapses are known as the "yo-yo" syndrome. In May of 2004, I decided to buy a special program known as Beachbody that looked very promising. It combined a daily one-hour exercise program and a diet program. I began the program weighing 135 pounds. By the end of August of 2004, I had lost a total of 19 pounds and my weight was an astonishing 116 pounds. Since then I have been able to maintain my weight between 112 and 117 pounds. You can find a program that can work very well for you. Just make sure that it is a healthy program and one that can become a way of life (daily regimen).

However, based on your age and health condition, consult with your primary care physician prior to starting this type of program.

I found that I needed to follow a program that teaches you how to eat healthy and exercise. Exercising alone and not combining it with a healthy diet will not give you the best results. The key here is to be consistent in order to be successful. Do not give up! You have to allow yourself attainable goals the same way that I did. For example, if your ultimate goal is to lose fifty pounds, do not concentrate on losing the fifty pounds at once. Instead concentrate on losing five pounds at a time in stages.

The other key is to eat with moderation and maintain a healthy diet. For example, stay away from fried foods. Just think that you deserve to eat healthy and to feel good! I do not claim to be an expert. I am just a normal person that has been able to accomplish something important in my life that can be attainable by anyone if done with consistency and the desire to do it as a way of life.

If your health is important to you, as it is for me, you can make positive changes and stick to them and not revert back to the old habits. Having the overall desire or need to follow a new "good" habit and finding enjoyment in doing so is the key, no matter what anyone else says. I used to visualize in my mind the way I wanted to look like, and that gave me the strength and motivation to continue in my goal. You can also look for a photo of when you were thinner and place it somewhere visible to give you the incentive to continue trying. I wrote an affirmation that I would read to myself everyday: "I love myself; therefore I deserve to be thinner and healthier." You can be your own leader and motivator! Just remember, life is a journey. Enjoy every step of your journey!

My Daily Supplements

The following are my daily supplements. The amounts depend on your condition and age. The younger you are, the less you need. For example, when I was under age fifty, I used to take 60mg of CoQ10. Presently I take 120mg of CoQ10 daily. As we age, the amount and potency should increase accordingly. Note: Consult with your doctor prior to taking some of these natural supplements if you are currently taking prescription medication.

As a result of my current lifestyle, not only do I have good health, but I also enjoy having lots of energy!

Product Name	Made By	Usage Instructions	Supplement Facts
Source of Life Gold Liquid Vitamins	Nature's Plus	1 capful per day	Used as a multivitamin, mineral and whole food liquid supplement
CoQ10 – 120mg	Pure Encapsulations	1 capsule per day	Used to improve cardiovascular system and circulation
Grape Pip – 500mg	Pure Encapsulations	1 capsule per day	Used as a potent antioxidant and supports vascular health
Biotin – 10,000mcg	Select a good brand	1 tablet per day	Used to promote healthy hair, nails and skin
Hair Essentials	Natural Wellbeing	3 capsules per day	Promotes hair growth
Apple Polyphenols	Apple Poly	1–2 capsules per day	Promotes hair growth, inhibits 5-alpha-reductase
Natural Joint	Greek Island Labs	1 capsule per day	Used to support healthy joint including join pain
Quercetin & Bromelain	Doctor's Best	2 capsules 2–3 times per day	Used for the treatment of eczema and allergies

Product Name	Made By	Usage Instructions	Supplement Facts
MSM – 1,000mg	Doctor's Best	1 or 2 capsules per day depending on need	Natural occurring sulfur helps the healing process of injuries and to detoxify the body on a cellular level
Dandelion Root – 525mg	Select a good brand	1 to 3 capsules per day depending on need	Acts as a diuretic for fluid retention. Cleanses the blood and liver and improves functioning of the kidneys, pancreas and stomach
Ultimate 10 Probiotic 30 billion	Vitamin Shoppe	1 or 2 capsules per day with food	Used to increase friendly bacteria in the stomach and intestines (10 strains)
OsteoBalance	Pure Encapsulations	7 capsules per day in divided dosages with food	Helps maintain healthy bones and bone density. Contains calcium plus other
Zinc – 50mg, Chelated	Select a good brand	1 capsule per day	Essential mineral. Helps with hairloss, high cholesterol, healthy immune system function and other
Poly-Gro Procyanidin B-2 (liquid)	Apple Poly	Shake well and apply twice daily to clean scalp and massage daily	Promotes hair growth. Inhibits 5-alpha-reductase

CHAPTER 4. MIND-SET

A positive mind-set, creating inner peace, eating healthy food, and practicing good habits can contribute toward obtaining good health. When one chooses to live in a positive and loving environment, life becomes easier. Our thoughts are more powerful than most of us realize. I believe that when we encounter a challenge, rather than dwelling on it, one should look for a solution. Sometimes solutions can be as simple as just changing our own viewpoint. We have no control over the way others think, but we can change the way we think.

Throughout my life, I have always been passionate about finding ways to stay healthy, to improve myself, and just learning how to play the game of life. I wanted to do well in all areas of my life and at least to be happy, that is, creating a good relationship with my family, including a successful marriage, doing well at work, and having personal satisfaction in whatever I choose to do. As a result of my research and experiences, I have come to the conclusion that our minds can contribute toward creating good health as well as poor health, besides what we eat. Our state of mind is reflected in our bodies depending on how we feel and what we are thinking. I have also read various books that have conveyed the same idea. Our health begins in our minds.

Coping with Stress

Let's talk a bit about stress. I describe stress as being the result of a lack of harmony in our state of mind. It is the result of someone's actions or situations, which are unpleasant to us or something that can cause great concern, whether at home or at work. For example, let's say you have a disagreement with your spouse or someone close to you—a family member or a friend at work. This occurrence can cause great discomfort. You could end up with a headache, an upset stomach, or any other uncomfortable outcome or stress. The best course of action is to confront the person you had the disagreement with. Communicate your feelings and resolve the disagreement in a loving way. However, what most people do is to take a pill to get rid of the headache or the upset stomach; maybe they just do not know what else to do? The only problem is that the source of the headache or upset stomach has not been addressed. It still exists and it can continue to cause discomfort in the future.

Whenever I feel stressed, I do the following breathing exercise: I go to a quiet area, stand with my legs apart, close my eyes, and extend my arms openly to my side. I then inhale deeply, at the same time bringing my arms with my palms open inward toward my chest. I then exhale slowly through my mouth and extend my arms outwardly away from my chest. This gives me a feeling of freedom. As I am doing this breathing exercise, I think of the following affirmation: "I breathe in peace and harmony. I exhale all stress." I visualize clean air coming in through my nose and a dark colored air coming out of my mouth. I keep doing this breathing exercise until I feel much better.

Always treat others with love, care, and respect, the same way you would like to have them treat you. By doing so, you would end up having fewer problems at work as well as unpleasant outcomes in your personal life. Here is a hypothetical situation: you are having a disagreement with an unreasonable individual with whom you cannot come to terms. Depending on your relationship with that person, if all attempts to resolve the issue fail, maybe the answer is to move on and disconnect from the source creating the unpleasant situation. If they don't respect you and want to abuse you, one needs to make a decision. Should I allow this to continue or should I free myself and get help? I went through a very tough experience and I disconnected and moved on. It was a very difficult chapter in my life being a single parent due to my divorce. I am so thankful I had my mother's support. I needed to heal from within. You've got to give yourself time to heal, love yourself, believe that you can get through it, and that you are strong. Try to read self-help and inspirational types of books. Take walks in the park; connect with the universe around you by admiring the beauty of trees, flowers, animals, children, and the elderly. Smile at them and be surprised how some will smile back even though they do not know you. Admire the sky, the sun, and feel the breeze touching your skin. If there is a lake close by, admire its beauty. I have done and experienced all this. By doing these things, your life can change for the better. Always have hope and never give up on yourself!

When dealing with family member disputes, you should try to resolve the disagreement as best as possible. Sometimes you may have to seek assistance from a neutral source such as a counselor. If this fails, you may have to keep a distance from them for a while until the condition of the situation subsides. At which point, you could try once more to open up communications with them and resolve the issue. Just remember, time only allows for the situation to ease up. However, it does not resolve the issues themselves. At the end of the day, the issues at hand usually will need to be confronted and resolved by coming to some form of mutual agreement.

Having a Positive Mind-set

Always remember we cannot change other people, but we have control of ourselves and the way we think. Just as our bodies need nutrition, so does our state of mind. That nutrition is a loving and peaceful environment where one can live in harmony with all around us.

The best formula for obtaining excellent results is having a "positive" mind-set, creating inner peace, and combining these with good habits, which include eating healthy, not smoking, and drinking minimum amounts of alcohol. When I was younger, I would drink one or two glasses of wine socially. At this point in my life, I have no desire to drink except maybe a bit when I go on vacation and on New Year's Eve. Your liver will love you when you minimize your alcohol consumption!

There are many books on the subject of how to live a good life and how to heal from within. These are just a few. I suggest you read any or all of the following:

The Secret by Rhonda Byrne
The Power by Rhonda Byrne
Think and Grow Rich by Napoleon Hill
You Can Heal Your Life by Louise L. Hay
Detoxification – A Clinical Doctor/Patient Manual by Dr. Richard Schulze

The Power of the Mind

I believe we become that which we believe to be. For example, as we grow older, if you have the preconceived notion of what you are supposed to look like at a certain age, then you can actually make this become a reality simply because you believe in it. If you have an unhealthy diet, your body will age faster as well.

Our mind is very powerful. It can create as well as destroy. The key is to know how to use it and always create good things. It takes a bit of practice and training.

I believe that for every action there is a result or a consequence, an outcome either good or bad. For example, if a person commits a robbery, that person will most likely experience a negative result by getting caught and being imprisoned. On the other hand, suppose you show extra care while performing a job for a client versus just getting the job done. The client was so appreciative of your work and caring attitude that not only did he pay you the agreed-to amount but also gave you a nice gift. This is a good and positive outcome. I believe that we have the power to decide which path to take in life. Life is full of options. However, no one can force you to do anything that you may consider to be unethical.

I believe that we are the product of our own thoughts. When you think positively, you attract positive things. For example, in the morning as I am driving to work, I look up to the sky and around me and say, "Thank you, God and the universe for another day of life. Today I am going to have a fantastic day! I will help my clients, I will make X amount of money. Thank you for my great husband! May he also have a great day. My son and the rest of my family have health and a good day as well!"

You can plan your day in your mind ahead of time. Make a decision that you will handle all things peacefully and without major stress.

Whenever you face adversity, remember that you may be dealing with other peoples' negative attitude, usually due to a problem. Others tend to thrive on negativity. They seem to always talk about negative things that have happened to them either at work or elsewhere, pulling their audience into their negative world. At the end of this conversation, the other participants also end up feeling in a very low state of mind. The important thing is to be strong and not to allow yourself to be affected by their toxic mind-set. Of course, it is easier said than done. However, by doing so, you may be able to help those individuals to feel better by giving them some kind of encouragement and helping them focus on finding a solution to their problem. However, if it is just trivial negative conversation, just change the subject to a more positive one.

As you become more focused on thinking positively and turning lemon situations into lemonade, life begins to turn around slowly and good things start to happen. At first you think it is just a coincidence, but as those coincidences occur more often, you begin to see a different picture. To give you an example, let's say you are looking for a parking space and cannot find one. Rather than getting upset, just think and say, "Someone will be leaving, and I am getting a parking space now."

The key is to issue a command, really believe in it, and it will happen. I do it all the time and my son tells me, "You really know how to get a parking space down pat, Mom." Some time ago, my son and I were in New York in an area quite difficult to find parking. We were in the car, double parked, and it took me about fifteen minutes to get parking. The car next to us was leaving, so I just backed up my car to let her leave and took the parking space. It really works! You need to have some patience with yourself until you learn how to do it. The more you practice, the easier it becomes. However, it works in any area of your life. You just make a command and believe that it will happen.

Let's suppose you need information or have a question you need an answer to. What you do is simply ask the question or state your request as if someone is listening to you. For example, just say, "I need to know *blank*; the answer is coming to me." Expect the answer; it does not matter how it comes, but it will come. You must believe it first, and then the answer will manifest itself usually from the least expected source. It is very cool how it works; the universe will answer you. It is amazing. I have experienced this several times. Coincidences do not exist. Most of the things that happen to us, we have something to do with creating them, even when we do not know we are actually doing it!

The "Spiritual" Side

I have always been in touch with my spiritual side. I believe that we are all connected spiritually. I also believe that there is a very powerful force, that although it is not visible to us, it does exist all around us. I believe that there is one creator, who is also referred to as God or divine power. This is a very powerful force that created us, and we are all connected to it. I believe that since we are all spiritual beings, our thoughts can be very powerful. I believe that we are also connected to the universe around us. Any creation begins with a thought. If you think and send a message of love and joy to the universe, you will receive that back. For example, make believe that you are making a phone call to someone and you leave a message of hate or bad wishes. What kind of a response would you most likely get back, a loving one or an angry response?

Just because you don't see this powerful force, it doesn't mean that it doesn't exist. Make your spiritual "phone call" to the universe and leave a message using a positive command. You will get your answer back. This may be in the form of an affirmation. For example, you can say, "I love myself; therefore I am ready to receive true love."

Mind Training

I believe that your mind must be kept active by exercising it in order to stay sharp and slow down the aging process. The same way we exercise our bodies to maintain health, our minds need it as well. There is a scientifically designed personalized training program on the web, which I think is fantastic for maintaining our brains in top shape. It is found on the web at www.lumosity.com. It is based on games that serve a purpose. There are various areas you would be working on to improve, such as your memory, attention, and problem solving. It is very well organized. It tracks your progress and is a lot of fun! I have been participating in this program for the past five years now. I can see the difference when I am actively doing it and when I am not. Try it; I am sure you will like it!

Final Thoughts

The idea of being at peace with everyone and being mentally free was always very important to me. One could say the following affirmation: "I release the need to hold on to old grudges. I forgive, therefore I am free."

I believe we should always be open to learn new things. This will give us the opportunity to grow and have a better life. I wrote this book with lots of love, with the desire to give you, my fellow reader, a message of hope that you can improve anything in your life!

MANUFACTURER AND DISTRIBUTOR INFORMATION

Below are the manufacturers and distributors of the brand-name products mentioned in this book.

Adonia Organics LLC
25 S Arizona Place
Chandler, AZ 85225
(800) 853-8840
www.adoniaorganics.com
Eye and skin care products.

Amazon.com, Inc.
410 Terry Avenue N
Seattle, WA
(206) 266-1000
www.amazon.com
Global merchandise distributor.

American Botanical Pharmacy
4114 Glencoe Ave
Marina Del Rey, CA 90292
(310) 821-2000
www.herbdoc.com
Organic herbal remedy products.

Aphogee
65 Shawmut Road STE 3
Canton, MA 02021
(855) 274-1313
www.aphogee.com
Hair care products.

Apple Poly LLC

303 Adams Ave Ste A

PO Box 732

Morrill NE 69358

(308) 247-3400

www.applepoly.com/healthyhair

Hair care products.

Arkopharma Laboratories (Migrastick)

BP 28 - 06511 CARROS Cedex – FRANCE

+33 (0)4 93 29 11 28

www.migrastick.com

Essential oils treatment for headaches.

Aztec Secret Health & Beauty LTD

P.O. Box 841

Pahrump NV, 89041

(775) 727-8351

www.aztec-secret.com

Skin care products.

Beachbody, LLC

3301 Exposition Blvd Fl 3

Santa Monica, CA, 90404

(800) 207-0420

www.beachbody.com

Fitness programs and nutritional supplements.

Beiersdorf Inc. (Eucerin - Aquaphor)

360 Dr Martin Luther King Jr. Dr

Norwalk, CT 06854-4655

(203) 563-5650

www.eucerinus.com

Skin care products.

Bobbi Brown Professional Cosmetics, Inc.
575 Broadway Fl 4
New York, NY, 10012
(646) 613-6500
www.bobbibrowncosmetics.com
Cosmetic products.

Doctor's Best, Inc.
197 Avenida La Pata Street
San Clemente CA 92673
(800) 333-6977
www.drbvitamins.com
Health nutritional supplements.

Dr. Bronner's Magic Soaps
1335 Park Center Drive
Vista, CA 92081
(844) 937-2551
www.drbronner.com
Body care products.

Enzymatic Therapy, Inc.
825 Challenger Drive
Green Bay, WI 54311
(800) 783-2286
www.enzymatictherapy.com
Health nutritional supplements.

Giovanni Cosmetics, Inc.
PO Box 6990
Beverly Hills, CA 90212
(310) 952-9960
www.giovannicosmetics.com
Hair and skin care products.

Good Hydrations (Phenomenal Water)
12383 Rough and Ready Hwy
Grass Valley, CA 95945
(800) 620-3365
www.phenomenalwater.com
Skin condition treatment products.

Greek Island Labs, LLC
7620 East McKellips Road Ste 4-86
Scottsdale, AZ 85257
(800) 449-6615
www.naturaljoint.org
Joint health supplements.

Juice Beauty
711 Grand Avenue Ste 290
San Rafael, CA 94901
(415) 457-4600
www.juicebeauty.com
Hair and skin care products.

Lumos Labs, Inc. (Lumosity)
140 New Montgomery Street, Fl 19
San Francisco, CA 94105
(877) 777-0502
www.lumosity.com
Online brain training and neuroscience research company.

Macy's, Inc.
7 West Seventh Street
Cincinnati, OH 45202
(513) 579-7000
www.macys.com
Major department store chain.

Mill Creek Botanicals
2951 Marion Drive #121
Las Vegas, NV 89115
(866) 447-6758
www.millcreekbotanicals.com
Hair and skin products.

Mirta de Perales, Inc.
2100 NW 96th Avenue
Doral, FL 33172
(305) 477-3703
www.mirtadeperales.us
Hair and skin care products.

MyChelle Dermaceuticals, LLC
1301 Courtesy Road
Louisville, CO 80027
(303) 228-7759
www.mychelle.com
Skin care products.

Natural Organics, Inc. (Nature's Plus)
548 Broadhollow Rd.
Melville, NY 11747
(631) 293-0030
www.naturesplus.com
Natural vitamins and nutritional supplements.

Natural Wellbeing Distribution Inc.
438 Westridge Parkway
Building 100
McDonough, GA 30253
(604) 733-2470
www.naturalwellbeing.com
Holistic Health Supplies and Remedies.

Neutrogena Corporation
5760 W 96th Street
Los Angeles, CA 90045
(310) 642-1150
www.neutrogena.com
Hair and skin care products.

NutriBullet, LLC
11755 Wilshire Blvd Ste 1200
Los Angeles, CA 90025
(855) 346-8874
www.nutribullet.com
Nutrition extractor.

Pure Encapsulations
490 Boston Post Road
Sudbury, MA 01776
(978) 443-1999
www.pureencapsulations.com
Nutritional supplements.

Roux (Colomer USA, Inc. Dist.)
5344 Overmyer Drive
Jacksonville, FL 32254
(904) 693-1200
www.rouxbeauty.com
Hair and skin care products.

Sally Beauty Supply, LLC
3001 Colorado Boulevard
Denton, TX 76210
(940) 898-7500
www.sallybeauty.com
Retail beauty supply chain.

Sun Chlorella USA
3305 Kashiwa Street
Torrance, CA 90505
(800) 829-2828
www.sunchlorellausa.com
Natural energy enhancing products.

The Hain Celestial Group, Inc. (Jason Powersmile Toothpastes)
1111 Marcus Avenue
Lake Success, NY 11042
(888) 659-7730
www.jason-personalcare.com
Personal care products.

The Vitamin Shoppe
2101 91st Street
North Bergen, NJ 07047
(201) 868-5959
www.vitaminshoppe.com
Natural vitamins and nutritional supplements.

Trader Joe's Company
800 S. Shamrock Avenue
Monrovia, CA 91016
(626) 599-3700
www.traderjoes.com
Specialty grocery store chain.

TYL Nutracueticals (Lydia Pinkham)

33 4th Street N. Ste 210

Petersburg, FL 33701

(727) 898.9668

www.lydiapinkham.org

Dietary supplement products for women.

Whole Foods Market, Inc.

550 Bowie Street

Austin, TX 78703

(512) 477-4455

www.wholefoodsmarket.com

Specialty grocery store chain.

3M Consumer Health Care Division (Buf-Puf)

2510 Conway Avenue

St. Paul, MN 55144

(800) 537-2191

www.bufpuf.com

Skin care products.

BIBLIOGRAPHY

Balch, Phyllis A. *Prescription for Nutritional Healing*. New York, NY: Penguin Group, 2006.

Byrne, Rhonda. *The Secret*. New York, NY: Atria Books, 2006.

———. *The Power*. New York, NY: Atria Books, 2010.

Hay, Louise L. *You Can Heal Your Life*. Carson, CA: Hay House Inc., 1994.

Hill, Napoleon. *Think and Grow Rich*. Seattle, WA: Pacific Publishing Studio, 2009.

Schulze, Richard. *Detoxification – A Clinical Doctor/Patient Manual*. Volume Two. Marina del Rey, CA: Natural Healing Publications, 2011.

ABOUT THE AUTHOR

I came to this land of opportunity on March 1, 1966, at the age of twelve. The day had finally arrived for my mother and me to leave Cuba. We only had a few pieces of clothing in an old suitcase. We went to the airport after saying goodbye to our family. Little did we know that we would never see them again, although my mother told them we would return in five years. At the airport, we were sitting in a large waiting room filled with chairs. Other people were also sitting there. All of us were hopeful that our names would be called so that we could board the plane bound for Florida, which meant freedom and a new life. Most people had been called and we were still there, afraid that we would have to go back home after having said goodbye to our family. I told my mother, "Don't worry I just know they are going to call our names," and sure enough they did! We were the last ones called on that day! A few other people had to go back home. We flew to Florida and stayed there for three days, then flew again with a new destination in New Jersey.

We lived for a month in the Carlton Hotel in Newark, New Jersey. My mother was able to find us an apartment in Union City, New Jersey, and acquired some used furniture and clothing through a local church.

I had dreams of going to school and becoming something big. My mother always said that if you have an education, doors will always open for you to create a better life for yourself and not have to depend on anyone. I struggled to learn the language.

I attended sixth grade at Edison Grammar School located in Union City. I only understood the math class; everything else was a big blur. It is so difficult when you want to understand what is being said and yet cannot due to the language barrier. However, I made many friends, and they were very helpful in translating for me.

I believe that if you set a goal, focus, and move toward it, you can achieve it. I told my mother that when I finished school and obtained a good job, I would help her pay our bills. My mother used to work in a factory in the garment industry. Her legs sometimes would become swollen and her knees would hurt. She still would continue to go to work regardless of how she felt. She was a very good-hearted, strong-minded woman and very spiritual. My mother was always there for me whenever I needed moral support. She was my best friend in addition to being a great mom. My mother was well liked by many people. Many of her friends would call her just to ask for her advice on many of their personal issues. She was very knowledgeable about life in general. Sadly, she passed away in July of 2013, four days short of her ninety-third birthday. It was a great loss for me, and I miss her very much. I always considered my mother as my role model and inspiration to go forward in life and never give up on myself.

In 1975, I was crowned Miss Union City in a local beauty pageant. I've had three careers in my lifetime. I graduated from Saint Peter's University in Jersey City, New Jersey with a bachelor's degree in accounting. I worked in accounting for twelve and a half years. I also worked as an investment counselor, having all the necessary licenses for fifteen years. Later, I went on to a new adventure by obtaining my cosmetology license and am currently working in the hair restoration industry.

I have learned that we must try our best to remain mentally positive even when we go through tough experiences like a bad marriage or a failed business. I went through both of these life experiences and believe me, both were very difficult! My first marriage ended in divorce. Thanks to my mom, who took care of my one-year-old son, I was then able to go to work without any worries. I was a single parent for many years. In May of 2000, I met my current husband, a wonderful man, via the Yahoo! Personal ads on the internet. In 2008, we were happily married after having a long engagement. My life has been quite a journey indeed!

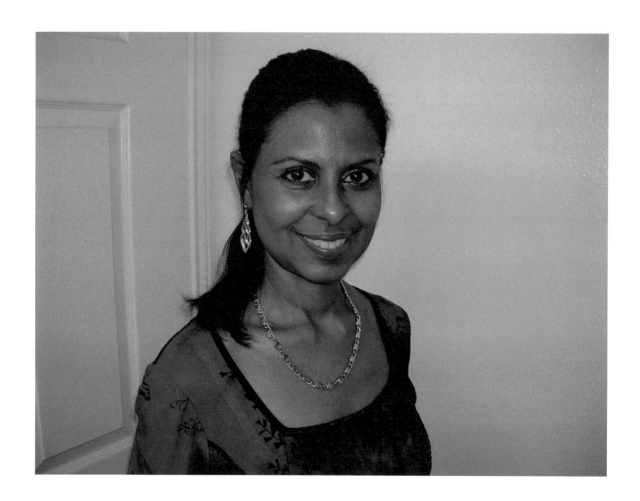

Printed in the United States
By Bookmasters